This Friendship Book belongs to:

....

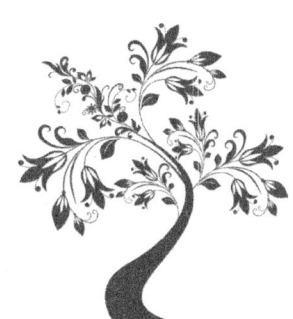

My motto:
Write it down now!

Stay on top of the news from friends and family!

When you see or talk to a friend or family member, take a few notes!

Jot down names, dates, events...

FRIENDSHIP *Book*

NAME: _____ **DATE:** _____
Met in person ☐　　Called ☐　　Messaged ☐
Key news:

Any follow-up needed?

NAME: _____ **DATE:** _____
Met in person ☐　　Called ☐　　Messaged ☐
Key news:

Any follow-up needed?

Did you promise to follow up in some way?

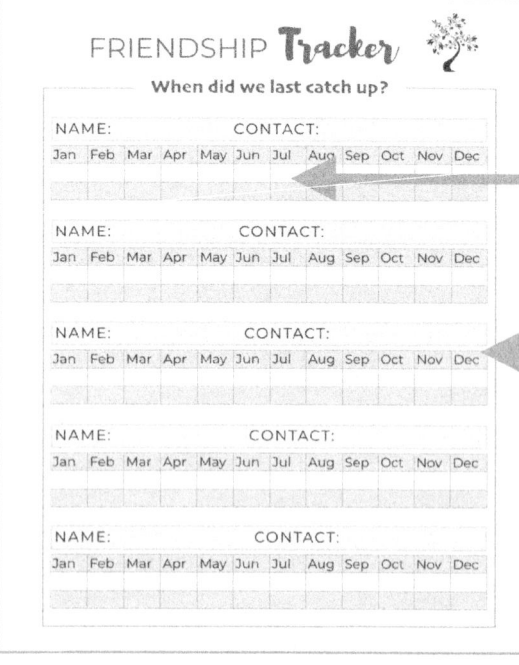

FRIENDSHIP *Tracker*
When did we last catch up?

NAME:				CONTACT:							
Jan	Feb	Mar	Apr	May	Jun	Jul	Aug	Sep	Oct	Nov	Dec

NAME:				CONTACT:							
Jan	Feb	Mar	Apr	May	Jun	Jul	Aug	Sep	Oct	Nov	Dec

NAME:				CONTACT:							
Jan	Feb	Mar	Apr	May	Jun	Jul	Aug	Sep	Oct	Nov	Dec

NAME:				CONTACT:							
Jan	Feb	Mar	Apr	May	Jun	Jul	Aug	Sep	Oct	Nov	Dec

NAME:				CONTACT:							
Jan	Feb	Mar	Apr	May	Jun	Jul	Aug	Sep	Oct	Nov	Dec

Then tick the box for this month in the friendship tracker at the front of the book.

The tracker will help you see when you last caught up – and if you really should get in touch!

Never forget those little details again!

There's also a month by month birthday and anniversary list... near the back of the book.

...so you never forget a happy (or a sad) day for a friend.

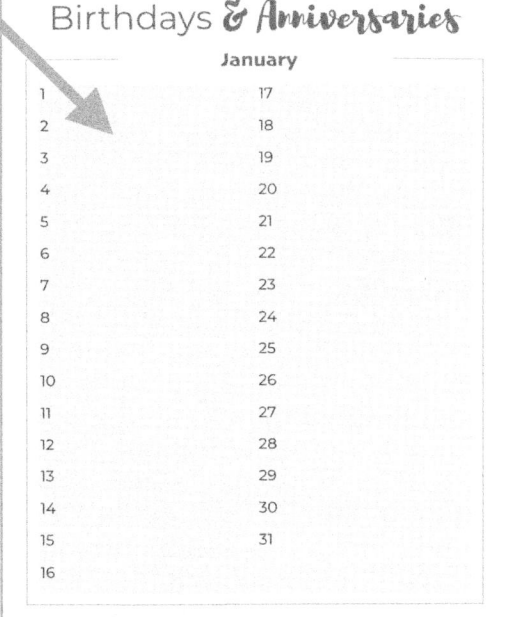

Birthdays & Anniversaries

January

1	17
2	18
3	19
4	20
5	21
6	22
7	23
8	24
9	25
10	26
11	27
12	28
13	29
14	30
15	31
16	

People in my life

NAME   SPECIAL THINGS

In appreciation of friends...

At the back of the book you'll find a 'special things' list to keep track of details like your friends' pet names or food preferences!

FRIENDSHIP *Tracker*

When did we last catch up?

NAME: CONTACT:

Jan	Feb	Mar	Apr	May	Jun	Jul	Aug	Sep	Oct	Nov	Dec

NAME: CONTACT:

Jan	Feb	Mar	Apr	May	Jun	Jul	Aug	Sep	Oct	Nov	Dec

NAME: CONTACT:

Jan	Feb	Mar	Apr	May	Jun	Jul	Aug	Sep	Oct	Nov	Dec

NAME: CONTACT:

Jan	Feb	Mar	Apr	May	Jun	Jul	Aug	Sep	Oct	Nov	Dec

NAME: CONTACT:

Jan	Feb	Mar	Apr	May	Jun	Jul	Aug	Sep	Oct	Nov	Dec

FRIENDSHIP *Tracker*

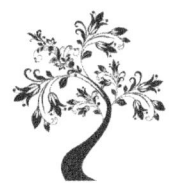

When did we last catch up?

NAME:				CONTACT:							
Jan	Feb	Mar	Apr	May	Jun	Jul	Aug	Sep	Oct	Nov	Dec

NAME:				CONTACT:							
Jan	Feb	Mar	Apr	May	Jun	Jul	Aug	Sep	Oct	Nov	Dec

NAME:				CONTACT:							
Jan	Feb	Mar	Apr	May	Jun	Jul	Aug	Sep	Oct	Nov	Dec

NAME:				CONTACT:							
Jan	Feb	Mar	Apr	May	Jun	Jul	Aug	Sep	Oct	Nov	Dec

NAME:				CONTACT:							
Jan	Feb	Mar	Apr	May	Jun	Jul	Aug	Sep	Oct	Nov	Dec

FRIENDSHIP *Tracker*

When did we last catch up?

NAME:				CONTACT:							

Jan	Feb	Mar	Apr	May	Jun	Jul	Aug	Sep	Oct	Nov	Dec

NAME:				CONTACT:							

Jan	Feb	Mar	Apr	May	Jun	Jul	Aug	Sep	Oct	Nov	Dec

NAME:				CONTACT:							

Jan	Feb	Mar	Apr	May	Jun	Jul	Aug	Sep	Oct	Nov	Dec

NAME:				CONTACT:							

Jan	Feb	Mar	Apr	May	Jun	Jul	Aug	Sep	Oct	Nov	Dec

NAME:				CONTACT:							

Jan	Feb	Mar	Apr	May	Jun	Jul	Aug	Sep	Oct	Nov	Dec

FRIENDSHIP *Tracker*

When did we last catch up?

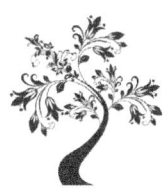

NAME:		CONTACT:									
Jan	Feb	Mar	Apr	May	Jun	Jul	Aug	Sep	Oct	Nov	Dec

NAME:		CONTACT:									
Jan	Feb	Mar	Apr	May	Jun	Jul	Aug	Sep	Oct	Nov	Dec

NAME:		CONTACT:									
Jan	Feb	Mar	Apr	May	Jun	Jul	Aug	Sep	Oct	Nov	Dec

NAME:		CONTACT:									
Jan	Feb	Mar	Apr	May	Jun	Jul	Aug	Sep	Oct	Nov	Dec

NAME:		CONTACT:									
Jan	Feb	Mar	Apr	May	Jun	Jul	Aug	Sep	Oct	Nov	Dec

FRIENDSHIP *Tracker*

When did we last catch up?

NAME:			CONTACT:								
Jan	Feb	Mar	Apr	May	Jun	Jul	Aug	Sep	Oct	Nov	Dec

NAME:			CONTACT:								
Jan	Feb	Mar	Apr	May	Jun	Jul	Aug	Sep	Oct	Nov	Dec

NAME:			CONTACT:								
Jan	Feb	Mar	Apr	May	Jun	Jul	Aug	Sep	Oct	Nov	Dec

NAME:			CONTACT:								
Jan	Feb	Mar	Apr	May	Jun	Jul	Aug	Sep	Oct	Nov	Dec

NAME:			CONTACT:								
Jan	Feb	Mar	Apr	May	Jun	Jul	Aug	Sep	Oct	Nov	Dec

FRIENDSHIP *Tracker*

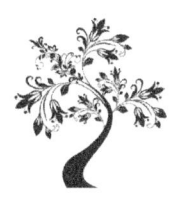

When did we last catch up?

NAME: CONTACT:

Jan	Feb	Mar	Apr	May	Jun	Jul	Aug	Sep	Oct	Nov	Dec

NAME: CONTACT:

Jan	Feb	Mar	Apr	May	Jun	Jul	Aug	Sep	Oct	Nov	Dec

NAME: CONTACT:

Jan	Feb	Mar	Apr	May	Jun	Jul	Aug	Sep	Oct	Nov	Dec

NAME: CONTACT:

Jan	Feb	Mar	Apr	May	Jun	Jul	Aug	Sep	Oct	Nov	Dec

NAME: CONTACT:

Jan	Feb	Mar	Apr	May	Jun	Jul	Aug	Sep	Oct	Nov	Dec

FRIENDSHIP Book

NAME:	DATE:

Met in person ☐   Called ☐   Wrote/messaged ☐

Key news:

Any follow-up needed?

NAME:	DATE:

Met in person ☐   Called ☐   Wrote/messaged ☐

Key news:

Any follow-up needed?

FRIENDSHIP Book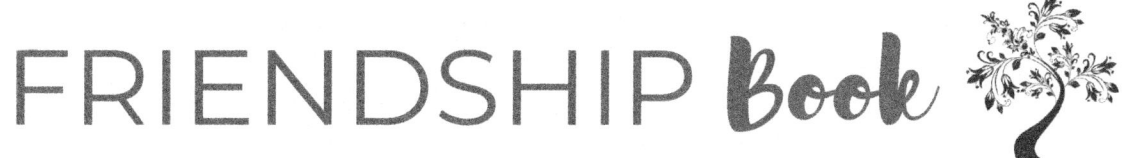

NAME:	DATE:

Met in person ☐ Called ☐ Wrote/messaged ☐

Key news:

....

....

....

Any follow-up needed?

◄───►

NAME:	DATE:

Met in person ☐ Called ☐ Wrote/messaged ☐

Key news:

....

....

....

Any follow-up needed?

FRIENDSHIP Book

NAME: | **DATE:**

Met in person ☐　　　Called ☐　　　Wrote/messaged ☐

Key news:

....

....

....

....

Any follow-up needed?

NAME: | **DATE:**

Met in person ☐　　　Called ☐　　　Wrote/messaged ☐

Key news:

....

....

....

....

Any follow-up needed?

FRIENDSHIP Book

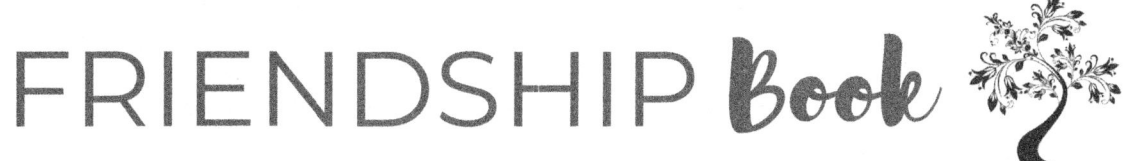

NAME: | **DATE:**

Met in person ☐　　　Called ☐　　　Wrote/messaged ☐

Key news:

....

....

....

Any follow-up needed?

NAME: | **DATE:**

Met in person ☐　　　Called ☐　　　Wrote/messaged ☐

Key news:

....

....

....

Any follow-up needed?

FRIENDSHIP *Book*

NAME: | **DATE:**

Met in person ☐   Called ☐   Wrote/messaged ☐

Key news:

....

....

....

Any follow-up needed?

NAME: | **DATE:**

Met in person ☐   Called ☐   Wrote/messaged ☐

Key news:

....

....

....

Any follow-up needed?

FRIENDSHIP Book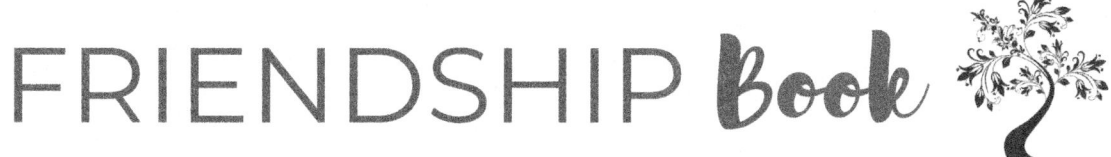

NAME: | **DATE:**

Met in person ☐   Called ☐   Wrote/messaged ☐

Key news:

Any follow-up needed?

NAME: | **DATE:**

Met in person ☐   Called ☐   Wrote/messaged ☐

Key news:

Any follow-up needed?

FRIENDSHIP *Book*

NAME: | **DATE:**

Met in person ☐   Called ☐   Wrote/messaged ☐

Key news:

....

....

....

....

Any follow-up needed?

NAME: | **DATE:**

Met in person ☐   Called ☐   Wrote/messaged ☐

Key news:

....

....

....

....

Any follow-up needed?

FRIENDSHIP *Book*

NAME: | **DATE:**

Met in person ☐   Called ☐   Wrote/messaged ☐

Key news:

....

....

....

Any follow-up needed?

NAME: | **DATE:**

Met in person ☐   Called ☐   Wrote/messaged ☐

Key news:

....

....

....

Any follow-up needed?

FRIENDSHIP Book

NAME: | **DATE:**

Met in person ☐ Called ☐ Wrote/messaged ☐

Key news:

Any follow-up needed?

NAME: | **DATE:**

Met in person ☐ Called ☐ Wrote/messaged ☐

Key news:

Any follow-up needed?

FRIENDSHIP *Book*

NAME: **DATE:**

Met in person ☐   Called ☐   Wrote/messaged ☐

Key news:

....

....

....

Any follow-up needed?

NAME: **DATE:**

Met in person ☐   Called ☐   Wrote/messaged ☐

Key news:

....

....

....

Any follow-up needed?

FRIENDSHIP Book

NAME: **DATE:**

Met in person ☐   Called ☐   Wrote/messaged ☐

Key news:

....

....

....

Any follow-up needed?

NAME: **DATE:**

Met in person ☐   Called ☐   Wrote/messaged ☐

Key news:

....

....

....

Any follow-up needed?

FRIENDSHIP Book

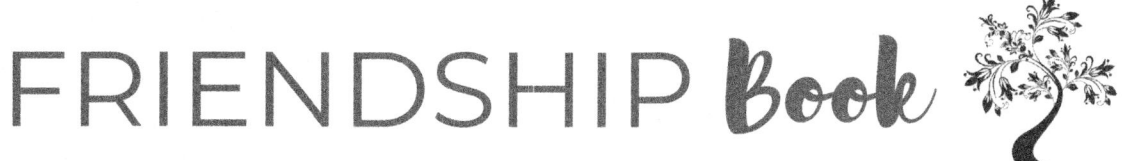

NAME:	DATE:

Met in person ☐   Called ☐   Wrote/messaged ☐

Key news:

Any follow-up needed?

NAME:	DATE:

Met in person ☐   Called ☐   Wrote/messaged ☐

Key news:

Any follow-up needed?

FRIENDSHIP *Book*

NAME: | **DATE:**

Met in person ☐   Called ☐   Wrote/messaged ☐

Key news:

Any follow-up needed?

NAME: | **DATE:**

Met in person ☐   Called ☐   Wrote/messaged ☐

Key news:

Any follow-up needed?

FRIENDSHIP Book

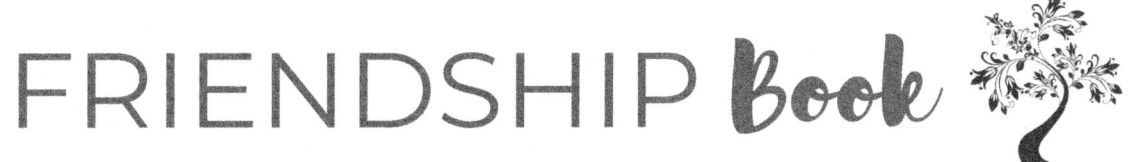

NAME: | **DATE:**

Met in person ☐   Called ☐   Wrote/messaged ☐

Key news:

Any follow-up needed?

NAME: | **DATE:**

Met in person ☐   Called ☐   Wrote/messaged ☐

Key news:

Any follow-up needed?

FRIENDSHIP *Book*

NAME: | **DATE:**

Met in person ☐　　Called ☐　　Wrote/messaged ☐

Key news:

....
....
....

Any follow-up needed?

NAME: | **DATE:**

Met in person ☐　　Called ☐　　Wrote/messaged ☐

Key news:

....
....
....

Any follow-up needed?

FRIENDSHIP Book

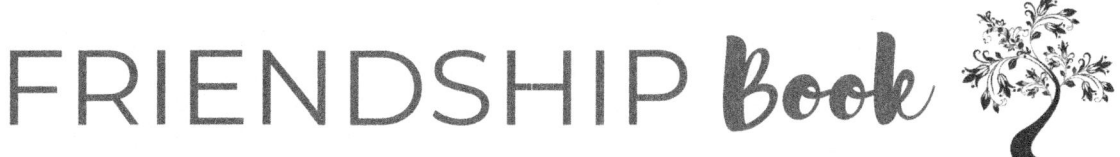

NAME: | **DATE:**

Met in person ☐   Called ☐   Wrote/messaged ☐

Key news:

....

....

....

Any follow-up needed?

NAME: | **DATE:**

Met in person ☐   Called ☐   Wrote/messaged ☐

Key news:

....

....

....

Any follow-up needed?

FRIENDSHIP Book

NAME: | **DATE:**

Met in person ☐　　　Called ☐　　　Wrote/messaged ☐

Key news:

Any follow-up needed?

NAME: | **DATE:**

Met in person ☐　　　Called ☐　　　Wrote/messaged ☐

Key news:

Any follow-up needed?

FRIENDSHIP *Book*

NAME: | **DATE:**

Met in person ☐   Called ☐   Wrote/messaged ☐

Key news:

Any follow-up needed?

NAME: | **DATE:**

Met in person ☐   Called ☐   Wrote/messaged ☐

Key news:

Any follow-up needed?

FRIENDSHIP *Book*

NAME:	DATE:

Met in person ☐   Called ☐   Wrote/messaged ☐

Key news:

....

....

....

Any follow-up needed?

NAME:	DATE:

Met in person ☐   Called ☐   Wrote/messaged ☐

Key news:

....

....

....

Any follow-up needed?

FRIENDSHIP Book

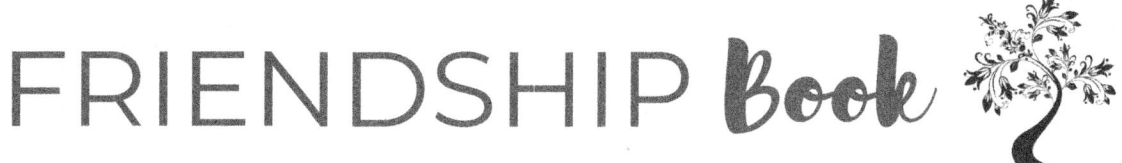

NAME:	DATE:

Met in person ☐   Called ☐   Wrote/messaged ☐

Key news:

....

....

....

Any follow-up needed?

NAME:	DATE:

Met in person ☐   Called ☐   Wrote/messaged ☐

Key news:

....

....

....

Any follow-up needed?

FRIENDSHIP Book

NAME: **DATE:**

Met in person ☐   Called ☐   Wrote/messaged ☐

Key news:

Any follow-up needed?

NAME: **DATE:**

Met in person ☐   Called ☐   Wrote/messaged ☐

Key news:

Any follow-up needed?

FRIENDSHIP Book

NAME: | **DATE:**

Met in person ☐   Called ☐   Wrote/messaged ☐

Key news:

Any follow-up needed?

NAME: | **DATE:**

Met in person ☐   Called ☐   Wrote/messaged ☐

Key news:

Any follow-up needed?

FRIENDSHIP *Book*

NAME: _____ **DATE:** _____

Met in person ☐ Called ☐ Wrote/messaged ☐

Key news:

....

....

....

....

Any follow-up needed?

NAME: _____ **DATE:** _____

Met in person ☐ Called ☐ Wrote/messaged ☐

Key news:

....

....

....

....

Any follow-up needed?

FRIENDSHIP Book

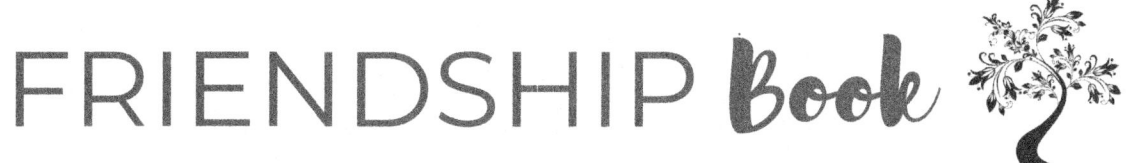

NAME: **DATE:**

Met in person ☐   Called ☐   Wrote/messaged ☐

Key news:

....

....

....

....

Any follow-up needed?

NAME: **DATE:**

Met in person ☐   Called ☐   Wrote/messaged ☐

Key news:

....

....

....

....

Any follow-up needed?

FRIENDSHIP Book

NAME: | **DATE:**

Met in person ☐   Called ☐   Wrote/messaged ☐

Key news:

....

....

....

Any follow-up needed?

NAME: | **DATE:**

Met in person ☐   Called ☐   Wrote/messaged ☐

Key news:

....

....

....

Any follow-up needed?

FRIENDSHIP Book

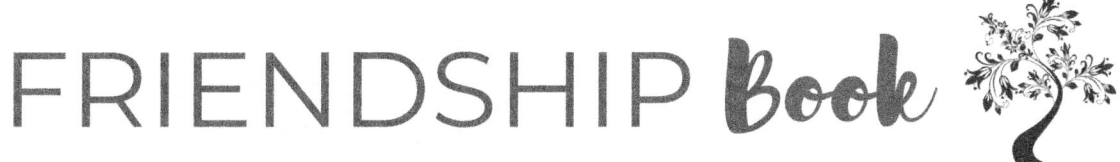

NAME: **DATE:**

Met in person ☐   Called ☐   Wrote/messaged ☐

Key news:

Any follow-up needed?

NAME: **DATE:**

Met in person ☐   Called ☐   Wrote/messaged ☐

Key news:

Any follow-up needed?

FRIENDSHIP Book

NAME: | **DATE:**

Met in person ☐ Called ☐ Wrote/messaged ☐

Key news:

....

....

....

....

Any follow-up needed?

NAME: | **DATE:**

Met in person ☐ Called ☐ Wrote/messaged ☐

Key news:

....

....

....

....

Any follow-up needed?

FRIENDSHIP Book

NAME: **DATE:**

Met in person ☐   Called ☐   Wrote/messaged ☐

Key news:

....

....

....

Any follow-up needed?

NAME: **DATE:**

Met in person ☐   Called ☐   Wrote/messaged ☐

Key news:

....

....

....

Any follow-up needed?

FRIENDSHIP *Book*

NAME: **DATE:**

Met in person ☐   Called ☐   Wrote/messaged ☐

Key news:

....

....

....

Any follow-up needed?

NAME: **DATE:**

Met in person ☐   Called ☐   Wrote/messaged ☐

Key news:

....

....

....

Any follow-up needed?

FRIENDSHIP *Book*

NAME:	DATE:

Met in person ☐   Called ☐   Wrote/messaged ☐

Key news:

Any follow-up needed?

NAME:	DATE:

Met in person ☐   Called ☐   Wrote/messaged ☐

Key news:

Any follow-up needed?

FRIENDSHIP *Book*

NAME:	DATE:

Met in person ☐   Called ☐   Wrote/messaged ☐

Key news:

....

....

....

....

Any follow-up needed?

NAME:	DATE:

Met in person ☐   Called ☐   Wrote/messaged ☐

Key news:

....

....

....

....

Any follow-up needed?

FRIENDSHIP *Book*

NAME: | **DATE:**

Met in person ☐   Called ☐   Wrote/messaged ☐

Key news:

....

....

....

Any follow-up needed?

NAME: | **DATE:**

Met in person ☐   Called ☐   Wrote/messaged ☐

Key news:

....

....

....

Any follow-up needed?

FRIENDSHIP *Book*

NAME:	DATE:

Met in person ☐   Called ☐   Wrote/messaged ☐

Key news:

Any follow-up needed?

NAME:	DATE:

Met in person ☐   Called ☐   Wrote/messaged ☐

Key news:

Any follow-up needed?

FRIENDSHIP *Book*

NAME: **DATE:**

Met in person ☐   Called ☐   Wrote/messaged ☐

Key news:

Any follow-up needed?

NAME: **DATE:**

Met in person ☐   Called ☐   Wrote/messaged ☐

Key news:

Any follow-up needed?

FRIENDSHIP *Book*

NAME: | **DATE:**

Met in person ☐ Called ☐ Wrote/messaged ☐

Key news:

Any follow-up needed?

NAME: | **DATE:**

Met in person ☐ Called ☐ Wrote/messaged ☐

Key news:

Any follow-up needed?

FRIENDSHIP *Book*

NAME: | **DATE:**

Met in person ☐ Called ☐ Wrote/messaged ☐

Key news:

Any follow-up needed?

NAME: | **DATE:**

Met in person ☐ Called ☐ Wrote/messaged ☐

Key news:

Any follow-up needed?

FRIENDSHIP Book

NAME: **DATE:**

Met in person ☐   Called ☐   Wrote/messaged ☐

Key news:

Any follow-up needed?

NAME: **DATE:**

Met in person ☐   Called ☐   Wrote/messaged ☐

Key news:

Any follow-up needed?

FRIENDSHIP Book

NAME:	DATE:

Met in person ☐   Called ☐   Wrote/messaged ☐

Key news:

Any follow-up needed?

NAME:	DATE:

Met in person ☐   Called ☐   Wrote/messaged ☐

Key news:

Any follow-up needed?

FRIENDSHIP *Book*

NAME:	DATE:

Met in person ☐   Called ☐   Wrote/messaged ☐

Key news:

....

....

....

....

Any follow-up needed?

NAME:	DATE:

Met in person ☐   Called ☐   Wrote/messaged ☐

Key news:

....

....

....

....

Any follow-up needed?

FRIENDSHIP Book

NAME:	DATE:

Met in person ☐　　　　Called ☐　　　　Wrote/messaged ☐

Key news:

....

....

....

Any follow-up needed?

NAME:	DATE:

Met in person ☐　　　　Called ☐　　　　Wrote/messaged ☐

Key news:

....

....

....

Any follow-up needed?

FRIENDSHIP *Book*

NAME: | **DATE:**

Met in person ☐   Called ☐   Wrote/messaged ☐

Key news:

Any follow-up needed?

NAME: | **DATE:**

Met in person ☐   Called ☐   Wrote/messaged ☐

Key news:

Any follow-up needed?

FRIENDSHIP Book

NAME: **DATE:**

Met in person ☐   Called ☐   Wrote/messaged ☐

Key news:

Any follow-up needed?

NAME: **DATE:**

Met in person ☐   Called ☐   Wrote/messaged ☐

Key news:

Any follow-up needed?

FRIENDSHIP *Book*

NAME:	**DATE:**

Met in person ☐   Called ☐   Wrote/messaged ☐

Key news:

....

....

....

Any follow-up needed?

NAME:	**DATE:**

Met in person ☐   Called ☐   Wrote/messaged ☐

Key news:

....

....

....

Any follow-up needed?

FRIENDSHIP Book

NAME: | **DATE:**

Met in person ☐   Called ☐   Wrote/messaged ☐

Key news:

Any follow-up needed?

NAME: | **DATE:**

Met in person ☐   Called ☐   Wrote/messaged ☐

Key news:

Any follow-up needed?

FRIENDSHIP *Book*

NAME: | **DATE:**

Met in person ☐   Called ☐   Wrote/messaged ☐

Key news:

....

....

....

Any follow-up needed?

NAME: | **DATE:**

Met in person ☐   Called ☐   Wrote/messaged ☐

Key news:

....

....

....

Any follow-up needed?

FRIENDSHIP Book

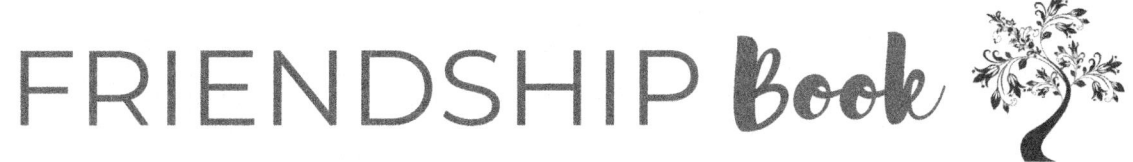

NAME:	DATE:

Met in person ☐　　　Called ☐　　　Wrote/messaged ☐

Key news:

Any follow-up needed?

NAME:	DATE:

Met in person ☐　　　Called ☐　　　Wrote/messaged ☐

Key news:

Any follow-up needed?

FRIENDSHIP *Book*

NAME: **DATE:**

Met in person ☐   Called ☐   Wrote/messaged ☐

Key news:

....

....

....

Any follow-up needed?

NAME: **DATE:**

Met in person ☐   Called ☐   Wrote/messaged ☐

Key news:

....

....

....

Any follow-up needed?

FRIENDSHIP *Book*

NAME:	DATE:

Met in person ☐   Called ☐   Wrote/messaged ☐

Key news:

....

....

....

Any follow-up needed?

NAME:	DATE:

Met in person ☐   Called ☐   Wrote/messaged ☐

Key news:

....

....

....

Any follow-up needed?

FRIENDSHIP Book

NAME:	DATE:

Met in person ☐   Called ☐   Wrote/messaged ☐

Key news:

Any follow-up needed?

NAME:	DATE:

Met in person ☐   Called ☐   Wrote/messaged ☐

Key news:

Any follow-up needed?

FRIENDSHIP *Book*

NAME:	DATE:

Met in person ☐   Called ☐   Wrote/messaged ☐

Key news:

....

....

....

....

Any follow-up needed?

NAME:	DATE:

Met in person ☐   Called ☐   Wrote/messaged ☐

Key news:

....

....

....

....

Any follow-up needed?

FRIENDSHIP *Book*

NAME:	DATE:

Met in person ☐   Called ☐   Wrote/messaged ☐

Key news:

....

....

....

....

Any follow-up needed?

NAME:	DATE:

Met in person ☐   Called ☐   Wrote/messaged ☐

Key news:

....

....

....

....

Any follow-up needed?

FRIENDSHIP Book

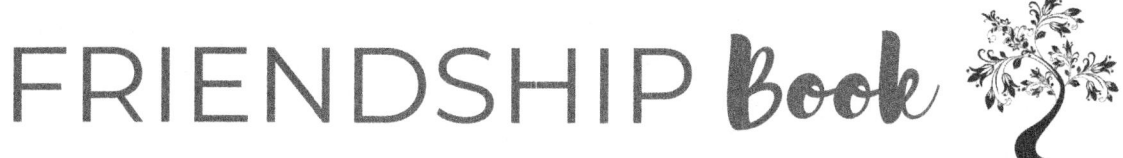

NAME: | **DATE:**

Met in person ☐   Called ☐   Wrote/messaged ☐

Key news:

....

....

....

Any follow-up needed?

NAME: | **DATE:**

Met in person ☐   Called ☐   Wrote/messaged ☐

Key news:

....

....

....

Any follow-up needed?

FRIENDSHIP *Book*

NAME:	DATE:

Met in person ☐   Called ☐   Wrote/messaged ☐

Key news:

Any follow-up needed?

NAME:	DATE:

Met in person ☐   Called ☐   Wrote/messaged ☐

Key news:

Any follow-up needed?

FRIENDSHIP Book

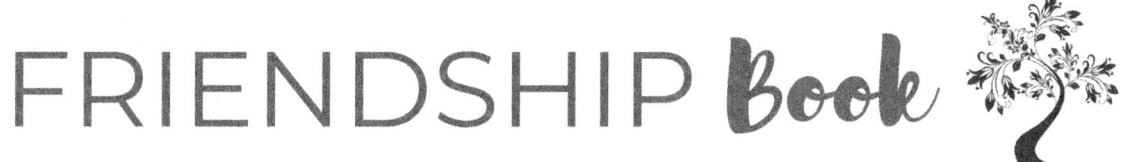

NAME: | **DATE:**

Met in person ☐ Called ☐ Wrote/messaged ☐

Key news:

Any follow-up needed?

NAME: | **DATE:**

Met in person ☐ Called ☐ Wrote/messaged ☐

Key news:

Any follow-up needed?

FRIENDSHIP Book

NAME: | **DATE:**

Met in person ☐   Called ☐   Wrote/messaged ☐

Key news:

Any follow-up needed?

NAME: | **DATE:**

Met in person ☐   Called ☐   Wrote/messaged ☐

Key news:

Any follow-up needed?

FRIENDSHIP Book

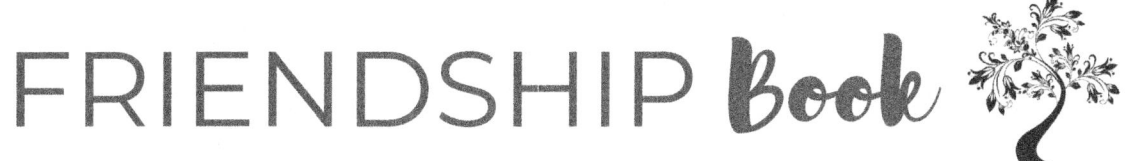

NAME:	DATE:

Met in person ☐   Called ☐   Wrote/messaged ☐

Key news:

....

....

....

Any follow-up needed?

NAME:	DATE:

Met in person ☐   Called ☐   Wrote/messaged ☐

Key news:

....

....

....

Any follow-up needed?

FRIENDSHIP Book

NAME: **DATE:**

Met in person ☐   Called ☐   Wrote/messaged ☐

Key news:

....

....

....

Any follow-up needed?

NAME: **DATE:**

Met in person ☐   Called ☐   Wrote/messaged ☐

Key news:

....

....

....

Any follow-up needed?

FRIENDSHIP *Book*

NAME:	DATE:

Met in person ☐   Called ☐   Wrote/messaged ☐

Key news:

Any follow-up needed?

NAME:	DATE:

Met in person ☐   Called ☐   Wrote/messaged ☐

Key news:

Any follow-up needed?

FRIENDSHIP *Book*

NAME:	DATE:

Met in person ☐   Called ☐   Wrote/messaged ☐

Key news:

Any follow-up needed?

NAME:	DATE:

Met in person ☐   Called ☐   Wrote/messaged ☐

Key news:

Any follow-up needed?

FRIENDSHIP Book

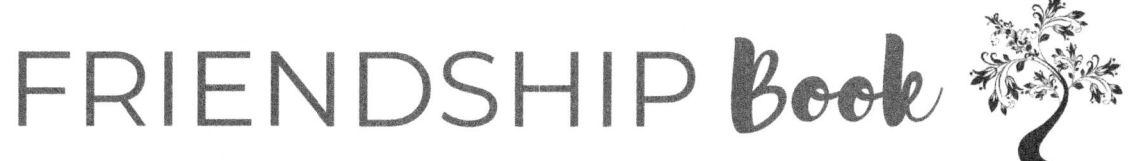

NAME:	DATE:

Met in person ☐   Called ☐   Wrote/messaged ☐

Key news:

....

....

....

....

Any follow-up needed?

NAME:	DATE:

Met in person ☐   Called ☐   Wrote/messaged ☐

Key news:

....

....

....

....

Any follow-up needed?

FRIENDSHIP Book

NAME: | **DATE:**

Met in person ☐   Called ☐   Wrote/messaged ☐

Key news:

Any follow-up needed?

NAME: | **DATE:**

Met in person ☐   Called ☐   Wrote/messaged ☐

Key news:

Any follow-up needed?

FRIENDSHIP Book

NAME: **DATE:**

Met in person ☐   Called ☐   Wrote/messaged ☐

Key news:

Any follow-up needed?

NAME: **DATE:**

Met in person ☐   Called ☐   Wrote/messaged ☐

Key news:

Any follow-up needed?

FRIENDSHIP *Book*

NAME: **DATE:**

Met in person ☐   Called ☐   Wrote/messaged ☐

Key news:

Any follow-up needed?

NAME: **DATE:**

Met in person ☐   Called ☐   Wrote/messaged ☐

Key news:

Any follow-up needed?

FRIENDSHIP Book

NAME: **DATE:**

Met in person ☐ Called ☐ Wrote/messaged ☐

Key news:

....

....

....

....

Any follow-up needed?

NAME: **DATE:**

Met in person ☐ Called ☐ Wrote/messaged ☐

Key news:

....

....

....

....

Any follow-up needed?

FRIENDSHIP Book

NAME:	DATE:

Met in person ☐ Called ☐ Wrote/messaged ☐

Key news:

Any follow-up needed?

NAME:	DATE:

Met in person ☐ Called ☐ Wrote/messaged ☐

Key news:

Any follow-up needed?

FRIENDSHIP Book

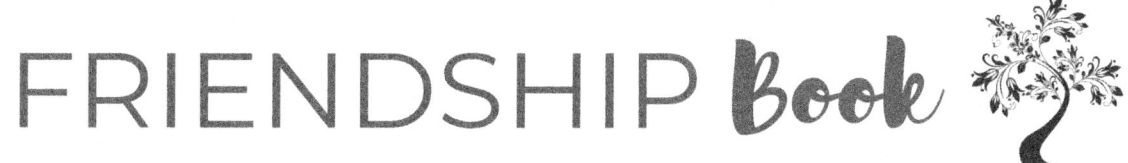

NAME: **DATE:**

Met in person ☐ Called ☐ Wrote/messaged ☐

Key news:

Any follow-up needed?

NAME: **DATE:**

Met in person ☐ Called ☐ Wrote/messaged ☐

Key news:

Any follow-up needed?

FRIENDSHIP Book

NAME:	DATE:

Met in person ☐   Called ☐   Wrote/messaged ☐

Key news:

Any follow-up needed?

NAME:	DATE:

Met in person ☐   Called ☐   Wrote/messaged ☐

Key news:

Any follow-up needed?

FRIENDSHIP *Book*

NAME: | **DATE:**

Met in person ☐   Called ☐   Wrote/messaged ☐

Key news:

....

....

....

Any follow-up needed?

NAME: | **DATE:**

Met in person ☐   Called ☐   Wrote/messaged ☐

Key news:

....

....

....

Any follow-up needed?

FRIENDSHIP *Book*

NAME: | **DATE:**

Met in person ☐   Called ☐   Wrote/messaged ☐

Key news:

....

....

....

Any follow-up needed?

NAME: | **DATE:**

Met in person ☐   Called ☐   Wrote/messaged ☐

Key news:

....

....

....

Any follow-up needed?

FRIENDSHIP *Book*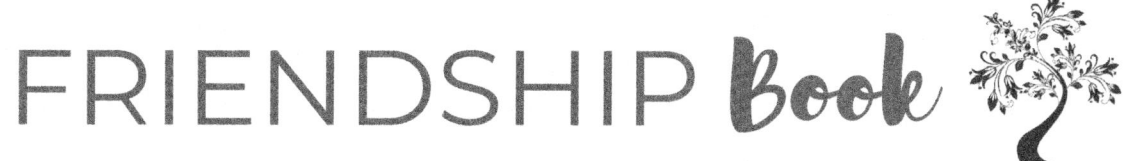

NAME: | **DATE:**

Met in person ☐   Called ☐   Wrote/messaged ☐

Key news:

....

....

....

Any follow-up needed?

NAME: | **DATE:**

Met in person ☐   Called ☐   Wrote/messaged ☐

Key news:

....

....

....

Any follow-up needed?

FRIENDSHIP Book

NAME:	DATE:

Met in person ☐ Called ☐ Wrote/messaged ☐

Key news:

Any follow-up needed?

NAME:	DATE:

Met in person ☐ Called ☐ Wrote/messaged ☐

Key news:

Any follow-up needed?

FRIENDSHIP Book

NAME:	DATE:

Met in person ☐   Called ☐   Wrote/messaged ☐

Key news:

....

....

....

....

Any follow-up needed?

NAME:	DATE:

Met in person ☐   Called ☐   Wrote/messaged ☐

Key news:

....

....

....

....

Any follow-up needed?

FRIENDSHIP *Book*

NAME: | **DATE:**

Met in person ☐   Called ☐   Wrote/messaged ☐

Key news:

....

....

....

....

Any follow-up needed?

NAME: | **DATE:**

Met in person ☐   Called ☐   Wrote/messaged ☐

Key news:

....

....

....

....

Any follow-up needed?

FRIENDSHIP Book

NAME:	DATE:

Met in person ☐   Called ☐   Wrote/messaged ☐

Key news:

Any follow-up needed?

NAME:	DATE:

Met in person ☐   Called ☐   Wrote/messaged ☐

Key news:

Any follow-up needed?

FRIENDSHIP *Book*

NAME:	DATE:

Met in person ☐   Called ☐   Wrote/messaged ☐

Key news:

....

....

....

Any follow-up needed?

NAME:	DATE:

Met in person ☐   Called ☐   Wrote/messaged ☐

Key news:

....

....

....

Any follow-up needed?

FRIENDSHIP Book

NAME: | **DATE:**

Met in person ☐　　　Called ☐　　　Wrote/messaged ☐

Key news:

....

....

....

Any follow-up needed?

NAME: | **DATE:**

Met in person ☐　　　Called ☐　　　Wrote/messaged ☐

Key news:

....

....

....

Any follow-up needed?

FRIENDSHIP *Book*

NAME:	DATE:

Met in person ☐   Called ☐   Wrote/messaged ☐

Key news:

Any follow-up needed?

NAME:	DATE:

Met in person ☐   Called ☐   Wrote/messaged ☐

Key news:

Any follow-up needed?

FRIENDSHIP Book

NAME: **DATE:**

Met in person ☐   Called ☐   Wrote/messaged ☐

Key news:

Any follow-up needed?

NAME: **DATE:**

Met in person ☐   Called ☐   Wrote/messaged ☐

Key news:

Any follow-up needed?

FRIENDSHIP *Book*

NAME:	DATE:

Met in person ☐   Called ☐   Wrote/messaged ☐

Key news:

....

....

....

Any follow-up needed?

NAME:	DATE:

Met in person ☐   Called ☐   Wrote/messaged ☐

Key news:

....

....

....

Any follow-up needed?

FRIENDSHIP *Book*

NAME:	DATE:

Met in person ☐   Called ☐   Wrote/messaged ☐

Key news:

....

....

....

....

Any follow-up needed?

NAME:	DATE:

Met in person ☐   Called ☐   Wrote/messaged ☐

Key news:

....

....

....

....

Any follow-up needed?

FRIENDSHIP *Book*

NAME: | **DATE:**

Met in person ☐　　　Called ☐　　　Wrote/messaged ☐

Key news:

....

....

....

....

Any follow-up needed?

NAME: | **DATE:**

Met in person ☐　　　Called ☐　　　Wrote/messaged ☐

Key news:

....

....

....

....

Any follow-up needed?

FRIENDSHIP Book

NAME: | **DATE:**

Met in person ☐ Called ☐ Wrote/messaged ☐

Key news:

Any follow-up needed?

NAME: | **DATE:**

Met in person ☐ Called ☐ Wrote/messaged ☐

Key news:

Any follow-up needed?

FRIENDSHIP *Book*

NAME: **DATE:**

Met in person ☐   Called ☐   Wrote/messaged ☐

Key news:

Any follow-up needed?

NAME: **DATE:**

Met in person ☐   Called ☐   Wrote/messaged ☐

Key news:

Any follow-up needed?

FRIENDSHIP *Book*

NAME:	DATE:

Met in person ☐　　　Called ☐　　　Wrote/messaged ☐

Key news:

....

....

....

Any follow-up needed?

NAME:	DATE:

Met in person ☐　　　Called ☐　　　Wrote/messaged ☐

Key news:

....

....

....

Any follow-up needed?

FRIENDSHIP *Book*

NAME: | **DATE:**

Met in person ☐   Called ☐   Wrote/messaged ☐

Key news:

Any follow-up needed?

NAME: | **DATE:**

Met in person ☐   Called ☐   Wrote/messaged ☐

Key news:

Any follow-up needed?

FRIENDSHIP Book

NAME: **DATE:**

Met in person ☐   Called ☐   Wrote/messaged ☐

Key news:

....

....

....

Any follow-up needed?

NAME: **DATE:**

Met in person ☐   Called ☐   Wrote/messaged ☐

Key news:

....

....

....

Any follow-up needed?

FRIENDSHIP Book

NAME:	DATE:

Met in person ☐　　　Called ☐　　　Wrote/messaged ☐

Key news:

....

....

....

....

Any follow-up needed?

NAME:	DATE:

Met in person ☐　　　Called ☐　　　Wrote/messaged ☐

Key news:

....

....

....

....

Any follow-up needed?

FRIENDSHIP Book

NAME: **DATE:**

Met in person ☐   Called ☐   Wrote/messaged ☐

Key news:

Any follow-up needed?

NAME: **DATE:**

Met in person ☐   Called ☐   Wrote/messaged ☐

Key news:

Any follow-up needed?

FRIENDSHIP *Book*

NAME:	DATE:

Met in person ☐   Called ☐   Wrote/messaged ☐

Key news:

....

....

....

....

Any follow-up needed?

NAME:	DATE:

Met in person ☐   Called ☐   Wrote/messaged ☐

Key news:

....

....

....

....

Any follow-up needed?

FRIENDSHIP Book

NAME:	DATE:

Met in person ☐   Called ☐   Wrote/messaged ☐

Key news:

....

....

....

....

Any follow-up needed?

NAME:	DATE:

Met in person ☐   Called ☐   Wrote/messaged ☐

Key news:

....

....

....

....

Any follow-up needed?

FRIENDSHIP *Book*

NAME: | **DATE:**

Met in person ☐ Called ☐ Wrote/messaged ☐

Key news:

....

....

....

....

Any follow-up needed?

NAME: | **DATE:**

Met in person ☐ Called ☐ Wrote/messaged ☐

Key news:

....

....

....

....

Any follow-up needed?

FRIENDSHIP Book

NAME: | **DATE:**

Met in person ☐   Called ☐   Wrote/messaged ☐

Key news:

....

....

....

Any follow-up needed?

NAME: | **DATE:**

Met in person ☐   Called ☐   Wrote/messaged ☐

Key news:

....

....

....

Any follow-up needed?

FRIENDSHIP Book

NAME:	DATE:

Met in person ☐   Called ☐   Wrote/messaged ☐

Key news:

....

....

....

Any follow-up needed?

NAME:	DATE:

Met in person ☐   Called ☐   Wrote/messaged ☐

Key news:

....

....

....

Any follow-up needed?

FRIENDSHIP Book

NAME:	DATE:

Met in person ☐   Called ☐   Wrote/messaged ☐

Key news:

Any follow-up needed?

NAME:	DATE:

Met in person ☐   Called ☐   Wrote/messaged ☐

Key news:

Any follow-up needed?

FRIENDSHIP Book

NAME:	DATE:

Met in person ☐   Called ☐   Wrote/messaged ☐

Key news:

....

....

....

....

Any follow-up needed?

NAME:	DATE:

Met in person ☐   Called ☐   Wrote/messaged ☐

Key news:

....

....

....

....

Any follow-up needed?

FRIENDSHIP *Book*

NAME: | **DATE:**

Met in person ☐ Called ☐ Wrote/messaged ☐

Key news:

....

....

....

Any follow-up needed?

NAME: | **DATE:**

Met in person ☐ Called ☐ Wrote/messaged ☐

Key news:

....

....

....

Any follow-up needed?

FRIENDSHIP *Book*

NAME:	DATE:

Met in person ☐ Called ☐ Wrote/messaged ☐

Key news:

Any follow-up needed?

NAME:	DATE:

Met in person ☐ Called ☐ Wrote/messaged ☐

Key news:

Any follow-up needed?

FRIENDSHIP Book

NAME: | **DATE:**

Met in person ☐ Called ☐ Wrote/messaged ☐

Key news:

Any follow-up needed?

NAME: | **DATE:**

Met in person ☐ Called ☐ Wrote/messaged ☐

Key news:

Any follow-up needed?

FRIENDSHIP *Book*

NAME: | **DATE:**

Met in person ☐   Called ☐   Wrote/messaged ☐

Key news:

....

....

....

....

Any follow-up needed?

───────────────────────────────────▶

NAME: | **DATE:**

Met in person ☐   Called ☐   Wrote/messaged ☐

Key news:

....

....

....

....

Any follow-up needed?

FRIENDSHIP Book

NAME: | **DATE:**

Met in person ☐ Called ☐ Wrote/messaged ☐

Key news:

....

....

....

Any follow-up needed?

NAME: | **DATE:**

Met in person ☐ Called ☐ Wrote/messaged ☐

Key news:

....

....

....

Any follow-up needed?

FRIENDSHIP *Book*

NAME: | **DATE:**

Met in person ☐ Called ☐ Wrote/messaged ☐

Key news:

Any follow-up needed?

NAME: | **DATE:**

Met in person ☐ Called ☐ Wrote/messaged ☐

Key news:

Any follow-up needed?

FRIENDSHIP *Book*

NAME:	DATE:

Met in person ☐   Called ☐   Wrote/messaged ☐

Key news:

....

....

....

Any follow-up needed?

NAME:	DATE:

Met in person ☐   Called ☐   Wrote/messaged ☐

Key news:

....

....

....

Any follow-up needed?

FRIENDSHIP Book

NAME: | **DATE:**

Met in person ☐ Called ☐ Wrote/messaged ☐

Key news:

....

....

....

Any follow-up needed?

NAME: | **DATE:**

Met in person ☐ Called ☐ Wrote/messaged ☐

Key news:

....

....

....

Any follow-up needed?

FRIENDSHIP *Book*

NAME:	DATE:

Met in person ☐   Called ☐   Wrote/messaged ☐

Key news:

....

....

....

Any follow-up needed?

NAME:	DATE:

Met in person ☐   Called ☐   Wrote/messaged ☐

Key news:

....

....

....

Any follow-up needed?

FRIENDSHIP *Book*

NAME:	DATE:

Met in person ☐   Called ☐   Wrote/messaged ☐

Key news:

....

....

....

....

Any follow-up needed?

NAME:	DATE:

Met in person ☐   Called ☐   Wrote/messaged ☐

Key news:

....

....

....

....

Any follow-up needed?

FRIENDSHIP Book

NAME:	DATE:

Met in person ☐   Called ☐   Wrote/messaged ☐

Key news:

Any follow-up needed?

NAME:	DATE:

Met in person ☐   Called ☐   Wrote/messaged ☐

Key news:

Any follow-up needed?

FRIENDSHIP Book

NAME:	DATE:

Met in person ☐　　　Called ☐　　　Wrote/messaged ☐

Key news:

....

....

....

Any follow-up needed?

NAME:	DATE:

Met in person ☐　　　Called ☐　　　Wrote/messaged ☐

Key news:

....

....

....

Any follow-up needed?

FRIENDSHIP Book

NAME: **DATE:**

Met in person ☐   Called ☐   Wrote/messaged ☐

Key news:

....

....

....

Any follow-up needed?

NAME: **DATE:**

Met in person ☐   Called ☐   Wrote/messaged ☐

Key news:

....

....

....

Any follow-up needed?

FRIENDSHIP Book

NAME: | **DATE:**

Met in person ☐ Called ☐ Wrote/messaged ☐

Key news:

Any follow-up needed?

NAME: | **DATE:**

Met in person ☐ Called ☐ Wrote/messaged ☐

Key news:

Any follow-up needed?

FRIENDSHIP Book

NAME:	DATE:

Met in person ☐   Called ☐   Wrote/messaged ☐

Key news:

....

....

....

....

Any follow-up needed?

NAME:	DATE:

Met in person ☐   Called ☐   Wrote/messaged ☐

Key news:

....

....

....

....

Any follow-up needed?

FRIENDSHIP *Book*

NAME:	DATE:

Met in person ☐   Called ☐   Wrote/messaged ☐

Key news:

....

....

....

Any follow-up needed?

NAME:	DATE:

Met in person ☐   Called ☐   Wrote/messaged ☐

Key news:

....

....

....

Any follow-up needed?

FRIENDSHIP Book

NAME:	DATE:

Met in person ☐   Called ☐   Wrote/messaged ☐

Key news:

Any follow-up needed?

NAME:	DATE:

Met in person ☐   Called ☐   Wrote/messaged ☐

Key news:

Any follow-up needed?

FRIENDSHIP *Book*

NAME:	DATE:

Met in person ☐   Called ☐   Wrote/messaged ☐

Key news:

....

....

....

Any follow-up needed?

NAME:	DATE:

Met in person ☐   Called ☐   Wrote/messaged ☐

Key news:

....

....

....

Any follow-up needed?

FRIENDSHIP *Book*

NAME:

DATE:

Met in person ☐   Called ☐   Wrote/messaged ☐

Key news:

Any follow-up needed?

NAME:

DATE:

Met in person ☐   Called ☐   Wrote/messaged ☐

Key news:

Any follow-up needed?

Birthdays & Anniversaries

January

1	17
2	18
3	19
4	20
5	21
6	22
7	23
8	24
9	25
10	26
11	27
12	28
13	29
14	30
15	31
16	

Birthdays & Anniversaries

February

1	17
2	18
3	19
4	20
5	21
6	22
7	23
8	24
9	25
10	26
11	27
12	28
13	29
14	
15	
16	

Birthdays & Anniversaries

March

1	17
2	18
3	19
4	20
5	21
6	22
7	23
8	24
9	25
10	26
11	27
12	28
13	29
14	30
15	31
16	

Birthdays & Anniversaries

April

1	17
2	18
3	19
4	20
5	21
6	22
7	23
8	24
9	25
10	26
11	27
12	28
13	29
14	30
15	
16	

Birthdays & Anniversaries

May

1	17
2	18
3	19
4	20
5	21
6	22
7	23
8	24
9	25
10	26
11	27
12	28
13	29
14	30
15	31
16	

Birthdays & Anniversaries

June

1

2

3

4

5

6

7

8

9

10

11

12

13

14

15

16

17

18

19

20

21

22

23

24

25

26

27

28

29

30

Birthdays & Anniversaries

July

1	17
2	18
3	19
4	20
5	21
6	22
7	23
8	24
9	25
10	26
11	27
12	28
13	29
14	30
15	31
16	

Birthdays & Anniversaries

August

1	17
2	18
3	19
4	20
5	21
6	22
7	23
8	24
9	25
10	26
11	27
12	28
13	29
14	30
15	31
16	

Birthdays & Anniversaries

September

1	17
2	18
3	19
4	20
5	21
6	22
7	23
8	24
9	25
10	26
11	27
12	28
13	29
14	30
15	
16	

Birthdays & Anniversaries

October

1	17
2	18
3	19
4	20
5	21
6	22
7	23
8	24
9	25
10	26
11	27
12	28
13	29
14	30
15	31
16	

Birthdays *& Anniversaries*

November

1	17
2	18
3	19
4	20
5	21
6	22
7	23
8	24
9	25
10	26
11	27
12	28
13	29
14	30
15	
16	

Birthdays & Anniversaries

December

1	17
2	18
3	19
4	20
5	21
6	22
7	23
8	24
9	25
10	26
11	27
12	28
13	29
14	30
15	31
16	

People in my life

NAME	SPECIAL THINGS

 In appreciation of friends…

People in my life

NAME	SPECIAL THINGS

In appreciation of friends…

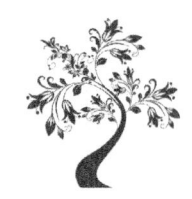

People in my life

NAME	SPECIAL THINGS

 In appreciation of friends…

People in my life

NAME	SPECIAL THINGS

In appreciation of friends...

Wishing you happy times with friends.

Printed in Great Britain
by Amazon

72237149R00081